The Healer's Way

Healing Professionals Share Inspiring Stories and
Proven Practices for Mind-Body Balancing

Curated by
Susana Perez

Table of Contents

INTRODUCTION

Welcome to "The Healer's Way," an extraordinary anthology that illuminates the transformative power of healing in its many dimensions. Within these pages, you will embark on a journey guided by an exceptional group of renowned healing experts whose wisdom and insights will inspire and empower you. As a bestselling author, Susana Perez is in awe of sharing this remarkable book and platform with these esteemed practitioners. Though not a healer herself, Susana recognizes the profound need to foster healing in our world and is passionate about bringing these transformative voices together.

In Chapter 1, Charlotte Larson invites us to discover the concept of Ikigai—a Japanese philosophy that uncovers our purpose and ignites joy in our existence. Moving forward, Constancia Gomez delves into the realm of intermittent fasting in Chapter 2, unveiling its potential to unlock profound health benefits, personal transformation, and empowerment.

Katie Wininger sheds light on Chapter 3, where the hidden truth of pain is unraveled, guiding us to explore its depths and find healing within. Chapter 4, authored by Kylee Alejandre, focuses on the healing journey during the postpartum period, offering insights and support to navigate this significant transitional phase.

In Chapter 5, Benjamin and Martina Jensen confront the profound issue of suicidality, reminding us that every life matters and shedding light on essential strategies for prevention and support. Michael Vanderplas presents a practical guide to mental health in Chapter 6, providing four transformative steps that lead to emotional well-being.

Naomi Haigh takes us on an introspective journey in Chapter 7, delving into the realms of self-discovery, personal growth, and the pursuit of fulfillment. Nathalie Herrey explores the life-changing power of gratitude in Chapter 8, illuminating how it can shift the trajectory of our lives and bring forth abundant blessings.

Regina Eco shares her wisdom in Chapter 9, unveiling the transformative potential of inner discovery through yoga—a practice that nourishes the mind, body, and soul. Sariah Boyer highlights the importance of touch for growth, healing, and the prevention of generational and physical trauma in Chapter 10.

Tina LeAnn Erdman introduces us to the fascinating world of Human Design in Chapter 11, an insightful tool that unravels the unique story of our individuality. Finally, in Chapter 12, Tina Jones empowers us to unlock the power of authenticity, guiding us toward a life of alignment, fulfillment, and self-expression.

"The Healer's Way" is a collection that encapsulates the diverse facets of healing, offering profound wisdom, empowering practices, and inspiring stories. Each chapter serves as a gateway to personal growth, inviting you to embark on your own transformative journey. Open your heart and mind as you explore the boundless possibilities of healing, and discover the path that resonates most deeply with your soul.

CHAPTER 1:
Ikigai: Finding Purpose and Joy in Life

The Japanese concept of *Ikigai* shines as a guiding light in our pursuit of a fulfilling and meaningful existence. Pronounced as "Icky Guy," Ikigai encompasses the profound sense of purpose that gives our lives direction and infuses them with passion and meaning. It represents the essence of what we live for and includes the unique combination of elements that bring us joy and fulfillment. Whether it is found in our work, relationships, hobbies, or contributions to the world, Ikigai is what we strive to achieve in this life.

Discovering our Ikigai is a deeply personal and ongoing journey that requires self-reflection, introspection, and exploration. It involves delving into our values, interests, talents, and aspirations to uncover the core motivations that drive us. As we navigate through the various stages of life, our Ikigai may evolve and transform, influenced by our experiences, personal growth, and shifting priorities. It is a dynamic concept that adapts to our ever-changing understanding of ourselves and the world around us.

Finding our Ikigai is not a one-time event but a continuous process of self-discovery. It invites us to explore our passions, aligns our actions with our values, and creates a sense of harmony between different aspects of our lives. The fluidity of Ikigai allows us to embrace change, adapt to new possibilities, and seize opportunities that may arise along our journey. It encourages us to remain open to new experiences, reevaluate our priorities, and adjust our path as we gain new insights and wisdom.

There may be days when our sense of purpose feels elusive or temporarily lost. It is important to remember that this is a natural part of the human experience. During these moments, we can employ various strategies to reconnect with our Ikigai and regain a sense of direction and fulfillment.

One such strategy is to stay mentally occupied with activities that bring us joy and a sense of accomplishment. It is up to each individual to determine what they genuinely enjoy doing. As long as we derive pleasure and fulfillment from our chosen activities, we can engage in them for the rest of our lives. This could involve pursuing a hobby, engaging in creative endeavors, contributing to a passionate cause, or simply immersing ourselves in activities that resonate with our interests and values. By finding joy and purpose in what we do, we infuse our lives with meaning and create a pathway to our Ikigai.

Efficiently utilizing time is another crucial aspect of embracing Ikigai. In today's fast-paced world, we often find ourselves caught in the trap of "hurry sickness," constantly rushing to accomplish short-term and long-term goals. However, the essence of Ikigai lies in building a harmonious relationship with time. Instead of being in a perpetual rush, we can learn to appreciate each moment and savor the present. By cultivating mindfulness and presence, we shift our perspective from a destination-oriented mindset to one that values the journey itself. This allows us to fully experience and appreciate the richness of life, fostering a deeper connection with our Ikigai.

Furthermore, cultivating meaningful relationships plays a vital role in our quest for Ikigai. Nurturing strong support systems encompassing family, friends, and social connections, contributes significantly to our overall well-being and sense of purpose. Investing time and effort into building and maintaining these relationships enhances our happiness and provides a sense of belonging and support as we navigate the challenges and triumphs of life.

Meaningful connections nourish our souls, provide the necessary encouragement and inspiration to pursue our passions and dreams and foster a sense of community that enriches our Ikigai journey.

It is essential to recognize that pursuing Ikigai is challenging. There will be moments when the path becomes arduous, and we may face obstacles or setbacks. However, it is during these trying times that our commitment to Ikigai is truly tested. We must embrace these challenges as opportunities for growth and transformation. Through adversity, we discover our resilience, learn valuable lessons, and deepen our understanding of ourselves and our Ikigai. The journey to Ikigai is not always smooth, but the rewards of living a purpose-driven life are immeasurable.

Living in alignment with our Ikigai not only brings personal fulfillment but also contributes to our overall well-being and happiness. When we have a sense of purpose and passion in our lives, we experience greater satisfaction and contentment. Studies have shown that individuals who have found their Ikigai tend to have lower stress levels, improved mental and physical health, and a higher quality of life. By nurturing our Ikigai, we create a positive ripple effect that extends to all areas of our lives and the lives of those around us.

Moreover, the journey to finding our Ikigai is not solely focused on personal gain. It is also about positively impacting the world and contributing to something greater than ourselves. When our actions are aligned with our Ikigai, we find meaning in serving others, whether it's through our work, volunteering, or supporting the causes we believe in. We create a purpose beyond personal fulfillment by using our unique talents and passions to benefit others.

Embracing Ikigai requires stepping out of our comfort zones and taking risks. It involves embracing the unknown, trying new things, and embracing failure as a stepping stone to growth. Through these experiences, we gain resilience, develop new skills, and broaden our perspectives. Each step taken on the Ikigai journey is an opportunity for self-discovery and self-improvement, leading us closer to a life of purpose and fulfillment.

In a world where we often prioritize productivity and external achievements, Ikigai reminds us of the importance of inner fulfillment and living a life in alignment with our deepest values and aspirations.

It calls us to reevaluate our priorities and make conscious choices that bring us closer to our true purpose. By regularly reflecting on our Ikigai, we can ensure that our actions and decisions align with our authentic selves.

In conclusion, Ikigai is a powerful concept that invites us to live a life of purpose, passion, and joy. It is a lifelong journey of self-discovery and alignment, where we continuously explore our desires, cultivate meaningful relationships, and utilize our time wisely. By embracing the challenges and uncertainties along the way, we gain resilience, grow as individuals, and contribute to a more meaningful and fulfilling existence. So, have you found your Ikigai? Let the search begin, and may your journey be filled with purpose, joy, and a profound sense of fulfillment.

About the Author

Charlotte Larson

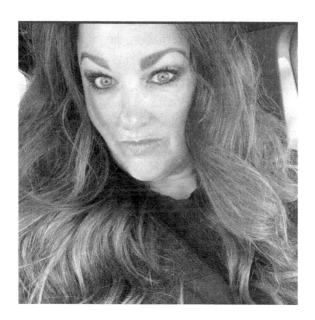

Charlotte Larson, the visionary behind True North Brain Center, is dedicated to empowering individuals in breaking free from the grips of the fight or flight mentality and achieving sustainable well-being. As the owner and driving force behind True North Brain Center, Charlotte has a comprehensive approach that combines cutting-edge techniques and compassionate guidance to help individuals reclaim their mental and emotional balance.

Her expertise in the field enables her to offer personalized strategies that address the unique needs of each client, guiding them toward a state of sustained harmony and resilience. As a resident of the vibrant community of Bountiful, Utah, Charlotte embodies the values of compassion, empathy, and community support. Her dedication extends not only to her clients but also to her family and pets, creating a nurturing environment that fosters growth and well-being for all.

For those seeking further information about Charlotte Larson and the services offered at True North Brain Center, an abundance of resources and insights await at https://www.truenorthbraincenter.com/. Delve into the expertise and passion that define Charlotte's work, and discover a path towards unlocking your true potential.

With Charlotte Larson at the helm, True North Brain Center serves as a beacon of hope and transformation, illuminating the way toward a life of vitality, peace, and lasting well-being.

CHAPTER 2:
Intermittent Fasting: Unlocking the Path to Health, Transformation, and Empowerment

Hola amigos! Constancia here, and I'm thrilled to have you join me on this extraordinary journey toward health, transformation, and empowerment through intermittent fasting. From a personal struggle with a cyst on my ovary to a groundbreaking discovery, intermittent fasting has profoundly impacted my life. In this comprehensive exploration, we will dive deep into the world of intermittent fasting, exploring its principles, remarkable benefits, real-life stories of transformation, and empowering practices that will propel you toward a healthier, happier you. So, grab a cozy seat and a refreshing beverage, and get ready to embark on a transformative adventure!

- A Quest for Optimal Health

Let's start our journey by delving into the origins of my pursuit of optimal health. A couple of years ago, when faced with a challenging cyst on my ovary, I committed to reclaim control over my well-being. This commitment set me on a path of exploration and research, leading me to discover the powerful concept of intermittent fasting. Intrigued and determined, I immersed myself in studying the science, philosophy, and practical applications of fasting as a means to enhance health and vitality.

- Demystifying Intermittent Fasting: A Flexible Approach

Now, let's demystify intermittent fasting and uncover its essence. Intermittent fasting is not a rigid diet but rather a flexible approach to nourishing our bodies. It involves cycles of eating and fasting, allowing us to tap into the body's innate ability to self-regulate and heal. I'll guide you through various fasting methods, such as time-restricted feeding, alternate-day fasting, and extended fasting, empowering you to find a fasting routine that aligns with your lifestyle and goals.

- Illuminating the Extraordinary Benefits

Prepare to be amazed as we explore the extraordinary benefits of intermittent fasting. Weight loss is just the tip of the iceberg. Through fasting, we activate a cascade of physiological processes that positively impact our health and well-being. We'll delve into the science behind improved insulin sensitivity, enhanced cellular rejuvenation, increased human growth hormone production, reduced inflammation, optimized brain function, lowered blood pressure and cholesterol levels, bolstered immune function, potential longevity benefits, and the psychological advantages of increased mental clarity, focus, and mindful eating habits.

- Cultivating Patience, Self-Love, and Mindset

Cultivating patience, self-love, and a positive mindset are crucial components of a successful fasting journey. Knowledge alone is not enough to sustain your progress. In this transformative process, it's essential to practice patience and understanding that lasting change takes time and consistency. Embracing self-love allows you to approach your fasting journey with compassion, kindness, and acceptance of yourself while nurturing a healthy relationship with your body and mind. Additionally, maintaining a positive mindset through affirmations, mindfulness techniques, and self-care practices helps you navigate challenges and stay committed to your fasting goals. By prioritizing these elements, you'll not only achieve physical transformations but also foster a profound sense of well-being and empowerment.

- My own experience

I have managed to lose 70 pounds thanks to my awesome discovery of intermittent fasting. I started to feel more energized and happy, plus I started to see the difference in my body, and my knees were happy. The weight I lost has shaped my life in some ways. Now I am taking charge of my health. Once I saw what it did for me, I started sharing what I knew.

One of my clients from my group, Anna, called me on an afternoon summer and was so happy that she needed to tell me all her news.

"I just came from the doctor and she is so happy with my results. My Doc mentioned that my cholesterol is better, and also, I was able to reduce my high blood pressure, and am no longer taking my pills for depression. So I wanted to really thank you for all your guidance and coaching, I couldn't have done it without your help."

- Wisdom from Fasting Experts

"Intermittent fasting is not a diet, it's a pattern of eating. It's a way of scheduling your meals so that you get the most out of them. It doesn't change what you eat, it changes when you eat." - Jason Fung, MD.

- Tailoring Your Fasting Journey

No two fasting journeys are the same, as we are all unique individuals with different lifestyles, preferences, and health considerations. This personalized approach will empower you to optimize the benefits of intermittent fasting while maintaining a balanced and sustainable lifestyle. One very important thing is to talk to your doctor, especially if you are taking medication. It's important to note that fasting may not be suitable for everyone, and it's essential to consult with a healthcare professional before starting any fasting regimen, especially if you have underlying health conditions or take medication.

- Embracing the Power of Community

The power of community and support cannot be underestimated on your fasting journey. Whether it's joining online forums, participating in accountability groups, or seeking guidance from healthcare professionals, connecting with like-minded individuals can provide encouragement, motivation, and a sense of belonging. That's why I created a group to support my clients.

- Your Journey Towards Empowerment Begins

Congratulations! You've reached the end of our comprehensive exploration of intermittent fasting. Armed with knowledge, inspiration, and practical tips, you are now ready to embark on your own transformative fasting journey. Remember, this is a personal voyage, and it's essential to listen to your body, be patient, and practice self-love along the way. As you embrace intermittent fasting, know that you have the power to take control of your health, transform your life, and become the empowered, vibrant, and radiant individual you were meant to be. ¡Adelante, mi amigo! Your journey towards health and transformation awaits.

About the Author

Constancia Gomez

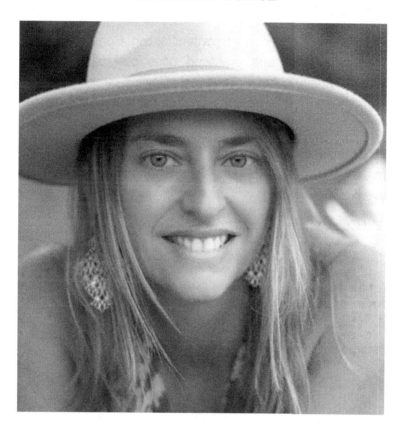

Constancia Gomez is a passionate advocate for conscious eating and intermittent fasting. She discovered the profound impact of essential oils in managing anxiety-related eating patterns, inspiring her to share her journey and empower others.

Alongside her writing endeavors, Constancia is a dedicated dancer, teacher, and author. Residing in Vermont with her partner, daughter, and their beloved animals, she finds solace and fulfillment on their farm.

Constancia's transformative journey began in 1999 when she arrived in the United States. Working at a ski resort in Vermont, she experienced shifts in her eating habits due to cultural differences and processed American foods. However, her passion for dance, especially tango, provided balance and helped her maintain a healthier weight.

Inspired by a live talk on intermittent fasting, Constancia embraced this lifestyle change and practiced conscious eating, leading to remarkable transformations. Today, she invites others to embark on their own health journeys, empowering them to make sustainable changes.

Constancia exemplifies the power of mindful choices and intermittent fasting, inspiring individuals to transform their lives and achieve well-being.

Find Constancia on Facebook

https://www.facebook.com/constanciagvt?mibextid=LQQJ4d

Youtube:

https://youtube.com/@constanciag.

Instagram:

https://instagram.com/constanciag?igshid=YmMyMTA2M2Y=

CHAPTER 3:
The Hidden Truth of Your Pain

Tears welled up and rolled down my cheek, "I don't know if depression is the right word. I don't want to be around anyone, I have to force myself to eat, I lie awake at night, I am getting migraines again, and my neck is so tense that I can't turn it in either direction." I had scheduled an emergency session with my therapist on a Monday afternoon; having experienced a falling out with a friend a few months prior, I was sure that's what this was about. After some digging, he pointed out, "So, it started around the time you decided to do foster care?" Whoa. Yes. How did I miss that? I was really excited to be a foster parent; at least, that's what I had been telling myself. I was so caught up in the chaos of getting the house ready and attending parenting classes that I wasn't allowing myself to slow down long enough to process any of it.

I am a seasoned professional when it comes to blowing off my body's subtle queues and emotions. I would have to get to the point of being completely overwhelmed, giving my brain no other option except to shut down all non-vital systems before I would listen. More common than you'd think, downplaying our negative emotions and avoiding spending time in our bodies might be contributing to prolonged physical symptoms.

The subconscious mind's job is to maintain homeostasis in the body, and its most effective form of communication is through physical sensations. We experience fatigue when we need to sleep and hunger when we need to eat; emotions are a basic process of life, so it makes sense that our subconscious mind would also have a way to signal something needing to be attended to there. Such as with the pain we may experience when we ignore subtle hunger queues, downplaying or outright ignoring emotions can actually make them worse. The subtle queues will likely get louder until they turn into screams for attention.

A study by The University of Texas at Austin in 2011 suggests that when emotions are bottled up, the person is more likely to act aggressively afterward. When you begin to think about this in relation to the physical sensations that are not being addressed, those angry outbursts might look closer to a pain flare-up or an autoimmune response.

According to Arthritis Foundation, "Multiple studies of osteoarthritis, rheumatoid arthritis, lupus and fibromyalgia show that people who experience more negative emotions also report more pain." The mind-body connection is more efficient than we give it credit for; instead of getting frustrated at the fact that we are feeling something, maybe we could try sitting with the pain and listening. While "All pain is generated in the brain," according to Dr. Howard Schubiner, "[it] is very real." Also, keep in mind that not all pain is psychological. Inflammation plays a role in the symptoms we experience from both physical injury and emotional pain; It's best to address both simultaneously.

In my early 20s, I was unaware of some unresolved trauma and would get debilitating migraines at least once a month. Migraines are a type of pain that demands a response. I would lay in an unlit room, ice pack in place while trying to will away the throbbing pain ripping through my head with each involuntary beat of my heart. After a few months in therapy, the migraines dissipated, I would only get them on occasion, and they were less debilitating. Then, I started working with a coach to address the migraines specifically.

I completely eradicated the migraines with a diet change cutting out all gluten and sugar temporarily, monthly massages, yoga, clearing out my negative emotions via the subconscious mind, and continuing to process my emotions as they come up. I'm not going to question which of these methods was the solution because it was likely all of them.

While all of the tools I implemented played a vital role for me, it's possible to see some progress without having to change your entire lifestyle. A client came to me when I was a new hypnotherapist; I wasn't yet confident that any of this would work. This client had an intense leg and foot pain from nerve damage related to diabetes, they were receiving acupuncture, pain injections, and massage.

After just one hypnosis session, they said they were completely out of pain. Their pain would slowly return between our sessions, but it got less intense each time. I regret not offering this client more – guiding them in clearing out their emotions or giving them some tips outside of our sessions. With that said, I want to offer you some of the tips and tools I have used on my own and with my clients.

First, allow yourself to ride the waves of emotion. According to Harvard Brain Scientist Dr. Jill Bolte Taylor, it takes ninety seconds to identify an emotion and allow it to dissipate while you simply notice it without judgment. When you try to investigate an emotion too soon, you may be talking yourself out of it, which can increase rumination and perseveration; In simple terms, you may be suppressing the emotion by trying to make sense of it.

Meditate, sit in silence, and ask yourself, "What am I feeling now?" feel the feelings and let them flow. Move your body; practice yoga, go on a walk in nature, dance around your living room, anything that gets your blood flowing and allows your body to move freely. Finally, see a therapist or a coach for an outside perspective. When I was sitting in my therapist's office, I couldn't see that becoming a foster parent was triggering past trauma and that I was terrified; he was able to observe what I wasn't seeing. Sometimes we get so embedded in the problem that we cannot see what it is actually about, and an outside perspective could make all the difference.

About the Author

Katie Wininger

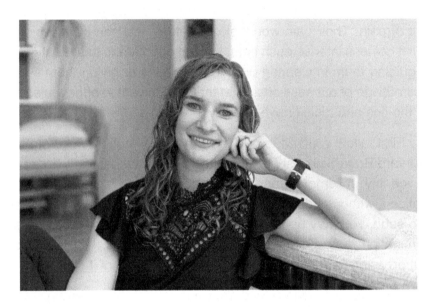

Katie Wininger is a Board Certified Hypnotherapist, Master NLP Coach, and Licensed Massage Therapist in the Wasatch Front Region of Utah. Coming from a traumatic background and growing up at the base of an almost 12,000 ft summit, the mountains have always been a welcomed stillness for Katie to explore her inner world. She loves almost all activities associated with them; just don't ask her to go BASE jumping. Katie started as a Massage Therapist in 2014, after years of concentrating on the physical symptoms of trauma and anxiety with her clients while simultaneously addressing her trauma. She could no longer deny that her clients needed more than she was able to give on the massage table. They needed to get to the root cause of their pain to make any real progress, just as she had done. Determined to find a solution for her clients, she became a coach in Neuro-Linguistic Programming. Now, in addition to massage, Katie supports her clients by exploring their subconscious patterns and then guiding them in clearing out suppressed emotions and unhelpful beliefs. When not playing in the mountains with her husband and dogs, you can find Katie at https://katiecoach.me/ or on Instagram @katie.wining

CHAPTER 4:
Healing in the Postpartum Period

In the United States, the average length of paid parental leave for someone who has given birth is twenty-nine days (1). A person is normally pregnant for about nine calendar months or forty weeks. During that time, the body is going through a plethora of changes. A expectant parent can experience a wide range of physical changes, such as weight gain, increased breast size, skin stretching, aches and pains, and so much more. Hormonal changes occur, as well, including an increase in progesterone and estrogen levels, which can lead to mood swings, fatigue, and nausea. Emotionally, pregnant individuals may experience heightened emotions, excitement, anxiety, and even depression. These are just a few examples of the many different symptoms that a expectant parent may experience, not to mention all of the discomforts, pains, and bodily changes that can occur during childbirth.

Keeping all of that in mind, it seems unbelievable that parents are expected to "bounce back" and return to their day jobs just twenty-nine days after giving birth. At the bare minimum, it takes six weeks for someone to recover physically from giving birth (2). That's not taking into account the emotional and hormonal recovery that needs to occur, which can take upwards of twelve to eighteen months following the birth.

Since parents are given so little time to recover from birth fully, it is even more important that certain steps are taken to optimize postpartum recovery and healing. Let's talk about a few of those steps.

Step One: Set boundaries and make a plan for visitors before the baby arrives.

Nothing is more draining on parents with a newborn than unwanted and/or unhelpful visitors. This is why it is crucial to decide whom you would like to have visit, when you will permit them to visit, and what you would like them to do while they are visiting. For instance, you may choose to have your mother stop by, but only after the baby is already two weeks old. Prior to her visit, it may be helpful to talk to your mother about how just holding the baby may not be what you need from her. You may need her to help with the dishes in the sink or throw a load of laundry in the washer prior to holding the baby. These can be difficult conversations to have with loved ones who are so excited to meet your baby, but they can also be crucial to getting your postpartum recovery started off on the right foot.

Step Two: Build a support team for the immediate postpartum period.

Many people are very fortunate to have family and friends who are available and happy to help with the twists and turns that come from having a baby and bringing that baby home. If you are one of those people, it is important to speak with your friends and family before your baby's arrival about a solid plan of support for you and your family after the baby has arrived. That plan should include meal support, housekeeping assistance, sibling care, pet care, etc.

On the other hand, if you do not have the support system that you would like to have available to you, it may be worth looking into hiring a postpartum doula. A postpartum doula is a professional trained in infant care and usually in infant feeding, so they can help you adjust to having a newborn. Postpartum doulas can also help you with anything that may be impeding you from bonding with your newborn and recovering from childbirth, including keeping up with housekeeping, meal preparation, sibling care, and so on. Enlisting the support of a postpartum doula is also great to do before the birth because doula support is something that you can usually add to a baby shower registry rather than a bunch of baby supplies that you may not even need.

Step Three: Rest, rest, rest.

While this may seem like an obvious follow-up to giving birth, it is often overlooked greatly in the postpartum period. When someone has a baby, they also expel the placenta, an organ that develops in the uterus during pregnancy and is responsible for providing nutrients and oxygen to the developing baby. When this placenta is released from the body minutes after the birth of the baby, it leaves behind a wound in the uterus that is about the size of a dinner plate. That wound takes about six weeks to heal fully, and that's only if the person who has given birth is getting plenty of rest over those six weeks. Without proper rest, that wound can take much longer to heal, which can lead to further complications. That's why it's so important to remember to prioritize rest in the immediate postpartum period and not rush the healing process, even if you feel like you are fully healed just a week after giving birth!

Step Four: Prioritize your nutrition.

It is so important to prioritize nutrition after having a baby because it supports physical postpartum recovery, provides essential nutrients for breastfeeding (if applicable), helps stabilize hormones, contributes to mood and mental health, supplies energy and stamina needed for childcare, strengthens the immune system, and aids in healthy weight management. A well-balanced diet during the immediate postpartum period supports the overall health of the person who has given birth, facilitates healing, and ensures optimal nourishment for both the parent and the baby. When planning for postpartum meals, it is very helpful to plan for sufficiently nutritious and well-balanced meals. If others are going to be helping you with meal preparation, it is also helpful to notify them in advance of your nutrition goals for optimal postpartum healing.

It is more important now than ever that your postpartum healing is taken seriously, especially in a country where it is not prioritized nearly enough in the professional world. The steps discussed here are just a few of the most important aspects of postpartum healing to consider, but healing needs can look different for each and every person. The most important thing to remember is to listen to your body and follow the cues that it is giving you. By acknowledging the significance of postpartum healing and prioritizing individual needs, we can create a supportive environment that values the well-being of those who have just given birth and fosters a healthier and happier start to the journey of parenthood.

References

1. Miller, C. C. (2021, October 25). The world "has found a way to do this": The U.S. lags on paid leave. The New York Times.

    https://www.nytimes.com/2021/10/25/upshot/paid-leave-democrats.html

2. Nguyen, H. (2023, March 27). Postpartum recovery: What to expect. HealthPartners Blog.

    https://www.healthpartners.com/blog/what-to-expect-after-giving-birth/

About the Author

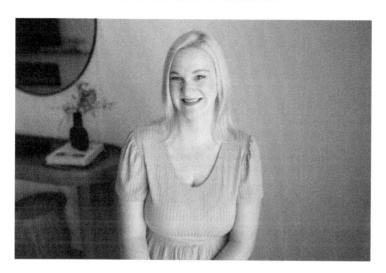

Kylee Alejandre is the owner of Doulas of Utah, https://doulasofutah.com/, a full-service doula agency in Northern Utah. Kylee is a certified birth doula, postpartum doula, placenta encapsulation specialist, and Hypnobabies childbirth educator. Throughout Kylee's own pregnancy, she learned just how much she didn't know about pregnancy and birth. Unfortunately, her first birth experience did not leave her with a strong sense of self-actualization or empowerment. She knew in her heart that the experience was meant to be one of great beauty, joy, and of course, strength. This led her to dig deeper into the research that surrounded birth. Through this research, Kylee stumbled across the topic of doulas and immediately began to immerse herself in this wonderful work. Since then, Kylee has supported countless families through pregnancy, birth, and the postpartum period. She is extremely passionate about this work, and she finds great joy in being a part of it. Kylee currently resides in Utah County with her loving husband, daughter, and mini-goldendoodle, and she is also awaiting the arrival of her second daughter.

CHAPTER 5:
Suicidality: One is Too Many

Throughout the history of time; Many people have had suicidal ideations. Many people have attempted suicide. Many people have successfully committed suicide. We can go into statistical numbers, what gender and race it affects most, but for anyone who has had suicide touch their lives, statistics don't matter. One is too high of a number to lose our loved ones to a preventable disease.

As a collective, we are tired of hearing the numbers and not having any action to support the suicidal population, and now we have a program that can help save those who suffer. What we have found from our research, listening to survivors, and stories from those who struggle with suicidal ideation is that no one really wants to die, they just want the pain to stop, and they don't know how to make it stop.

If you haven't been in that disparity, it's hard to comprehend. Suicidality is one of those taboo topics we're afraid of speaking up, afraid of not speaking up, and in reality, we're just scared we're going to push the suicidal person over the edge, and then how do we cope when the person is successful? Or that people will criticize us if they find out that we failed to stop them. The other problem we see is that someone says they're suicidal, but in reality, they are seeking attention. If someone is really doing it for attention, there is something they're in need of, too, and that needs to be addressed as well. So it is better to show support to everyone and be proactive in getting them help than to try to determine who is qualified to get treatment or not.

Many special days/months are set aside for suicide awareness but very little talk about the healing process of suicidal ideations. There are more programs for grieving people who have lost their loved ones to suicide than those who struggle with suicidality. Why is that? We believe that because of the complexity of suicidality, we cannot continue to treat this disease as a singular modality, but instead, it needs to be addressed through multiple modalities and include a complete spectrum approach including physical, mental, emotional, spiritual, and community. When we're looking at the well-being of a individual, we have to look at the whole person, not just one aspect. We can potentially miss the activating or triggering event by looking at a single aspect.

Humans can be generally covered by looking at the physical, mental, emotional, and spiritual aspects of their lives. You have to SEE them as a whole and not separate them into aspects, as that will affect the other aspects. For example, if you have catastrophizing or ruminating thoughts this can trigger emotional reactions such as anxiety, stress, anger, depression, etc. If you have an emotional or spiritual stressor, this can trigger those same negative thoughts and also, in turn, manifest physically. This looks like pain, sickness, and inability to perform tasks.

To properly treat any person, you have to look and see that person as a whole, or you will miss the who, what, how, and why of what they are dealing with. YOU WILL NOT SEE THEM until you see all of them. How can we help those in a suicidal crisis? People who are in crisis cannot properly problem solve, and need assistance in their decision making regarding their necessities. They don't know what they need; they can't think about little things. You will have to be the one to take over for them. You need to make sure they're eating nutritious food. You have to be the one to give them commands or ask direct questions. An example may be saying, "Come on, we're going for a walk." As you say this, you reach for their hand and guide them on the walk. You should ask them questions like, "Is this helping?" or "Are you feeling any different," if the answer is yes, ask, "Good different or bad different?" if it's good, continue; if it is bad to ask, "what doesn't feel good?" and adjust accordingly. Be very specific, we're looking for the small things that help; big and complex things will be too overwhelming. While the standard 'make a safety plan' with them is not a bad thing, there are other things that can help more. Staying with them so they're not alone; at the minimum, use the guide below.

1. Validate their feelings; it doesn't matter if you understand or not, these are their feelings, and they're real to them.

2. Physical contact brings them back to their body instead of being stuck in their heads.

3. Guided earthing/grounding helps them come back to their body, too, and grounding especially helps regulate their system overall.

4. Be their mental and emotional guide; as we mentioned above, they cannot think for themselves; they are malfunctioning in many different body systems.

The journey doesn't stop here. The need for community support (a village) is the foundation needed to continue further healing and stability for those who have suffered. In essence, this is a re-birth, a new cycle, a new support, a new beginning.

Author's note: I had a village, and I conquered the darkness that controlled me, in contrast to my brother who did not have a village, who did not reach out for help because he didn't know what he needed, and the darkness took him. It truly takes a village and to be seen as whole to overcome the darkness and pain. May the future be: Many people have conquered their suicidal ideations. Many people have conquered treatment. Many people have LIVED.

About the Authors

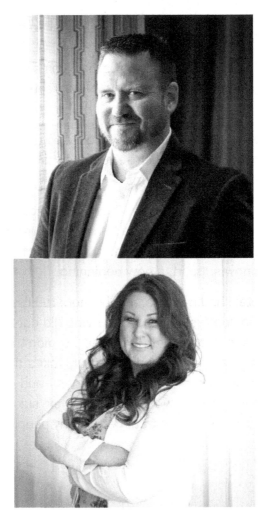

Benjamin Jensen MA, CMHC (Masters in Clinical Mental Health Counseling, Bachelor's of Health Science). Martina Jensen BS, AAS (Bachelor of Health Science, Associate of Applied Science, Nanotechnology). Benjamin and Martina met in prison.... (as correctional officers). Since then, they have been pushing each other to reach their highest potential, which landed them back at school together. They both earned their bachelor's of health science, and Ben received his master's degree in clinical mental health counseling. Together they own Roots & Meadows https://www.rootsandmeadows.com/, which focuses on getting to the root cause of the ailments, not just covering up the symptoms, and using the most natural modalities possible. After losing Martina's brother to suicide and Martina being a suicide survivor herself, they knew there needed to be a program to help those who suffer from suicidal ideations, not just to mask the symptoms. They looked at all the differences between the two situations and designed a program to fit the needs of those who are in disparity. In their free time, they enjoy traveling, gardening, biking, rock hounding, revitalizing old homes, and other adventures with their children.

CHAPTER 6:
4 Easy Steps to Mental Health

I remember thinking, "Are many of my patient's sad, angry, afraid because they are sick, or are they sick because they are sad, angry, and afraid?" I realized that throughout my entire career, I had been looking at the problem the wrong way. If I could help them early to heal their mind, emotions, and soul, maybe I could prevent the negative epigenetic results of thoughts and feelings on their physical bodies. If I could do that, maybe I could help keep people out of hospitals by providing healthy and happy living.

Your behaviors, environment, and what you mentally and emotionally focus on affect your risk of illness. For millennia, ancient texts have taught these principles. Luckily, with recent developments in neuroscience, we know that many of these ideas are backed by hard, evidenced science. With that in mind, let's focus on the three stay pools that create positive mental health.

Identity, Connection, Direction:

We are social beings. It sounds nice, but it's also INCREDIBLY true. Our need to be around other people is deeply embedded in our DNA. For most of our existence as a species on this planet, life has been brutal. Our daily goal was simply not to get sick, killed by a predator, and find enough food to live to the next day. No stores to buy food. No "social-media" to retreat to pseudo-interactions with others. We literally developed the NEED to connect with others, and that connection program still runs in us.

By interacting as an integral part of a small, 25–150-person tribe, each one of us knew who we were and our role to ensure the survival of our tribe and ourselves. We were certain of our identity with others.

Our direction was simply: to survive. The need for Identity, Connection, and Direction still subconsciously runs in our everyday behaviors.

But what is our Identity, Connection, and Direction today? Even though it's easy to get food, shelter, and safety today, those original programs are still ingrained in us. However, the ease of modern-day physical survival is also what has produced mental and emotional problems that are so prevalent today. Those things that came to us instinctively (the need for Identity, Connection, and Direction to survive) are the things that we are searching for today on a different level. The good news is we can find them hidden in our unconscious mind.

Carl Jung said, "until you make the unconscious, conscious, it will direct your life and you will call it fate."

Our modern-day goal is to make the unconscious conscious and discover our individual Identity, develop healthy connections, and discover our life's direction. It's a life-long goal, yet by following these four simple steps, what is unconscious will slowly rise to the surface and become clear to each one of us.

4 Steps Daily

Years ago, I felt massively depressed, like life had no purpose. I didn't know who I was. I felt distant from everyone—negative thoughts filled every second of my waking mind. If I could get just one moment of distraction, that would be one minute of peace. I wanted time to figure it out. Unfortunately, I had to do survival things like make money so I could buy food. I wanted to avoid people at work but had to interact with them from time to time.

But work got in the way. As an ICU nurse, I sometimes needed to look up and study difficult concepts. I had to lift and reposition my patients throughout the day. Sometimes a coworker would say something funny as we worked.

One day I realized that when I was focused on all the aspects of my work, I wasn't focused on all the stuff going on in my life. I found my one minute of peace. The strategy had simply evolved unconsciously. All I had to do now was to realize what steps I had unconsciously taken to give me the peace I was looking for.

I came across four common tasks that I was practicing. I further realized that if I engaged in these daily that the negative thoughts seldom snuck in.

1. Physical

Neuroscientists have pointed out that what we do has a far greater result on our mental health than trying to think our way out of a rut. It's incredibly difficult to control our minds with our minds. When your mind is not where you want it to be, use the body to shift the mind. When you do, you will shift the chemicals that are released in your brain, which will allow you to regain control of your mental steering wheel.

Take a walk. Workout. Do yard work, do housework, or just focus on your breathing. Whatever it is, physical action changes your mindset.

2. Intellectual

The most incredible thing about us humans is that we can envision the future. With this unique ability comes the inner-driven desire to be and know more. When we engage in learning something new, we calm our minds. So read a book. Watch a documentary. Talk to someone smarter than yourself. When we do something intellectual, we feel better about ourselves.

3. Work

There is a sense of accomplishment when we do something. Carl Jung stated, "You are what you do, not what you say you'll do." It's the actions that we complete which define our identity.

Taking steps towards completing something unpeels the layers of who we believe ourselves to be until we reach the core of who we truly are. Do some writing. Volunteer with a group or an organization. Put something together from IKEA. Maybe just go to your job and work. It could distract you from negative thoughts. You might even discover who your innermost self is too.

4. Social

As stated above, we NEED social interaction. If you need to improve at connecting with others, remember social skills are like muscles. The more we exercise them, the stronger they become.

Ask a friend to dinner. Go out to a sporting event or art show. Take a hike. Even if you are alone, you can tell the other people on the trail to have a nice day. Chances are they will tell you the same.

About the Author

Michael Vanderplas

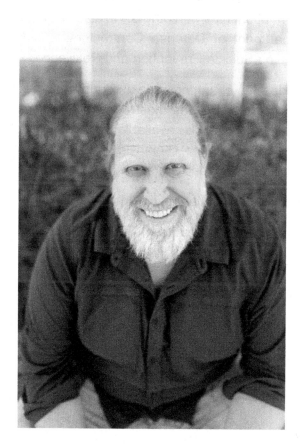

Michael is a complete healer. As an ICU and Psychiatric Nurse for over two decades, Michael has been in more life-and-death situations than most. This has given him incredible insight into the total life spectrum. Having flown over 1,000,000 miles, his public speaking and trainings have taken him to Australia, Brazil, Canada, El Salvador, Germany, Guatemala, Mexico, and the Netherlands. In a lifelong quest to improve himself and those around him, in 2017, he completed a long-time goal to become a Master Trainer of Hypnosis and NLP.

In 2022 he became an International best-selling author with his debut book "Stay Strong – Overcome Suicidal Thoughts and Live the Life You Always Wanted."

Michael currently works daily with active-duty military helping them overcome past and present traumas, build resilience, and form healthy relationships with others. He also has advised the U.S. Military, Department of Defense Contractors, and NATO Allied Forces regarding Suicide Prevention and Resilience.

He provides life-changing breakthrough coaching as well as group trainings that utilize the most advanced unconscious mind-mapping assessment tools available today. He also provides certification training in Hypnosis, NLP (Neuro-Linguistic Programming), and Suicide Awareness.

You can contact him via the information below.

www.enlightened-academy.com

YouTube: Viking Nurse @vikingnurse4319

Instagram: mike_vanderplas

Facebook: https://www.facebook.com/Michael.Vanderplas.NLP

Email: vanderplasmike25@gmail.com

CHAPTER 7:
Finding Your Inner Truth

I discovered I was a Medium at the ripe age of 37. Up until that point, there were no prominent signs. I never considered myself "spiritually gifted" before then. I did feel like I saw the world a lot differently than my peers, but I couldn't describe how it was different, only that I felt like there was more to life than what we were seeing with our eyes every day. As is usually the case, my soul was onto something that my brain wasn't quite comprehending.

This has been a continuous lesson from the Universe since stepping into my calling as a Medium, Psychic, Healer, Teacher, and Human. Our souls know ALL the answers we are seeking! And I was, and still am, always seeking more truth! Before my spiritual awakening, as most of us in the spiritual community call it, I relied heavily on my logic and intelligence. I went through Business school and got what I thought, at the time, was my dream job. I was a Business Analyst for a bank holding company that owned seven national banks. I got the corporate job, the fancy title, a corporate credit card, set my own schedule, mainly worked remotely, got to travel, and all the perks! But I was still seeking. There was something that I was "missing" in all of this. Something I wasn't quite seeing. I was like Neo from The Matrix, searching for something that was looking for me.

And when I found it, I found out it was ME. I put ME in capital letters for a reason. It wasn't little Naomi Haigh me; it was soul ME. So, my journey began to find out what that meant. I started by learning about *Reiki*. Reiki is the Japanese form of energy healing which includes energetically balancing out the *chakras*, the main energy points in your body. This was the first time I was ever introduced to any sort of energy healing, and the experience I had left me wanting to know everything about it that I could. I found a teacher and started learning about energy, meditation, healing, the Universe, connections to spirit, and more.

As I started practicing Reiki on others, that's when my Mediumship started opening up. I felt a presence enter the room, but I could not see it. My clairaudience was strong, which came in the form of hearing words in my head as I was working on people. The words would guide me to different parts of the person's body that wanted attention. I found a few other mentors to teach me how to strengthen my Mediumship skills, then found I was naturally attuned to helping others learn what their gifts were and help them strengthen them. I learned I could use my gifts in Business, as well. That is a highlighted version of my spiritual awakening and journey, but I will now dive into the work it takes to be able to access these amazing gifts! Ready to hear it?!

"Awakening is not changing who you are, but discarding who you are not." – Deepak Chopra.

This is the HOW, my friends! This is how you seek those answers within. A spiritual awakening/journey comes with learning your own unique process of questioning your current beliefs and learning which ones really, deeply hold true to your soul. This process of questioning what you believe to be true, which can range in beliefs as far and wide as your heart desires, is the way to clear up the unwanted inner noise to listen to the peaceful, inner voice that is your soul. You can start with a certain area of your life to keep things simple. For example, think of what you believe about your own spirituality.

If you want to commune with energy and spirits, ancestors, guides, etc., this is a foundation that needs to be established to do that. Are your beliefs set in stone and certain, or are there some gray areas where you aren't quite sure where you stand on some things? If you're set in stone, think about where that belief came from and check in with your heart to see if that feels expansive or if it feels like you've convinced yourself because you've adopted someone else's belief. If there are some gray areas, then that shows that there is still truth you can seek within and start sitting with yourself and asking those questions, then see what naturally comes up for you. This is how you build your intuition.

You take the time to sit with yourself, ponder your beliefs and feelings, and then let your body and soul help guide you to discovering YOUR truth. If it's true for you, it will feel expansive and warm; you might hear a "YES" internally or many other iterations of similar feelings. That is your soul speaking to your mind and telling you it aligns with that belief. You keep those and use those beliefs as your foundation.

This process can get ugly. I say ugly because there's usually some ugly crying involved! You know, the crying where the eyes swell like biscuits, the snot runs, and crazy ungodly noises escape your mouth. Don't be afraid of that, though. It's clearing out all the mistruths, which is necessary and way past due! You are getting to the bottom of your basement, where all the forgotten boxes and maybe stale, rotted food has been sitting for months, years, or most likely decades. It needs to come out. Then you can lay down new beliefs, the kind that empowers you, that light you up. The beliefs you WANTED to believe in the first place. The beliefs that bring you back to oneness with yourself, with each other, and with the world around you. You are perfect. You are whole. You are needed. You are worthy. You are supported. You are loved! You are loved! You are loved!

About the Author

Naomi Haigh

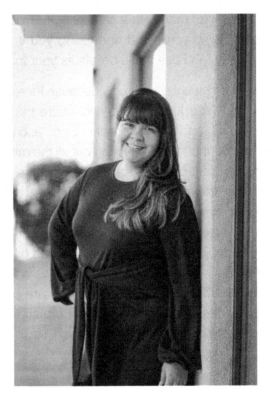

Naomi Haigh is a multi-talented individual, bridging the realms of spirituality and business with finesse. As a Psychic Medium, Business Consultant, Energy Healer, and Teacher, she brings a unique blend of insights and wisdom to her work.

Not content with keeping her knowledge to herself, Naomi takes the role of a guiding light through her captivating podcast, The Modern Psychic Podcast. With each episode, she fearlessly dives into what it truly means to be a psychic in today's world. Through her expert guidance, she offers diverse pathways for listeners to tap into their innate psychic abilities and seamlessly integrate them into their everyday lives and professional ventures.

Educated at USU, Naomi holds an impressive academic background, boasting an MBA and Masters in Human Resources. This comprehensive education equips her with a deep understanding of the intricacies of business and the human element within it.

Beyond her professional pursuits, Naomi cherishes her role as a devoted spouse and a proud mother of two incredible sons. Their presence fuels her passion and serves as a reminder of the boundless potential of love and connection.

With her expansive skill set and genuine commitment to empowering others, Naomi Haigh stands as a beacon of inspiration, illuminating the way for individuals seeking to embrace their spiritual gifts while excelling in the world of business.

CHAPTER 8:
Gratitude Will Change Life's Trajectory

G ratitude is a powerful emotion that has a profound impact on our lives. When we practice gratitude, we are acknowledging the good things in our lives and express appreciation for them. This simple act of gratitude positively changes the trajectory of our lives in many ways.

Firstly, gratitude improves our mental health. When we focus on the positive things in our lives, we are less likely to dwell on negative thoughts and emotions. This reduces stress and anxiety and improves our overall mood. Studies have shown that people who practice gratitude regularly have lower levels of depression and anxiety, sleep better, and are more resilient in the face of adversity. I personally call the practice of gratitude a superpower - and who doesn't want one of those?!

Secondly, gratitude improves our relationships with others. When we express gratitude towards others, we strengthen our bonds with them and build trust and intimacy. Gratitude also inspires us to be more generous and compassionate towards others, which can further improve our relationships. Research has shown that people who express gratitude towards their partners have more positive interactions and feel more satisfied in their relationships.

Thirdly, gratitude improves our physical health. When we are grateful, we are more likely to engage in healthy behaviors such as exercising, eating well, and getting enough sleep. Gratitude also boosts our immune system and reduces inflammation in the body, which can reduce the risk of chronic diseases such as heart disease and diabetes. As we become older, this becomes more and more important.

Finally, gratitude improves our overall sense of well-being and happiness. When we focus on the good things in our lives, we are more likely to feel content and satisfied. Gratitude also helps us to feel more connected to others and to something larger than ourselves, which gives our lives a sense of purpose and meaning. I have personally found that as I have gotten more fluid in the 'attitude of gratitude,' I am more likely to see things to be grateful for. Every day has miracles.

So how can we practice gratitude in our daily lives? Here are some simple strategies:

1. Keep a gratitude journal – Write down three things you are grateful for each day. Don't overwhelm yourself; 3 things are plenty as you start out! It can be as simple as you being grateful for your toothbrush or bed, for example. This will help you to focus on the positive things in your life and cultivate a sense of gratitude.

2. Express gratitude towards others – Take the time to thank someone for something they have done for you. This can be as simple as thanking your partner for doing the dishes or thanking a colleague for their help on a project. I can promise as you do this as a practice, the world will seem more positive and kinder.

3. Practice gratitude during difficult times – When you are facing a challenging situation, try to find something to be grateful for. This helps you to shift your perspective and find hope and positivity in the midst of adversity. I remember a friend of mine telling me that whenever she thought life was hard, she would think of me and my life, and she would feel better - that is a silver lining, if any! And I was, in a way, grateful that my life, and my trials, were able to make her stronger in hers.

4. Practice mindfulness – Take the time to be fully present and pay attention to the small moments of joy and beauty in your life. This helps you to cultivate a sense of gratitude and appreciation for the present moment. Don't forget that sleep is an essential part of practicing mindfulness.

In conclusion, gratitude is a powerful emotion that positively changes the trajectory of our lives. By practicing gratitude regularly, we can improve our mental and physical health, strengthen our relationships with others, and increase our overall sense of well-being and happiness. So take the time to cultivate gratitude in your daily life and see how it can transform your world. As you do, I would love to hear about how those transformations affect your life because I know it will open up a whole new way of experiencing life and, most importantly - happiness.

References

https://news.harvard.edu/gazette/story/2017/04/over-nearly-80-years-harvard-study-has-been-showing-how-to-live-a-healthy-and-happy-life/

https://www.cnbc.com/amp/2023/02/10/85-year-harvard-study-found-the-secret-to-a-long-happy-and-successful-life.html

https://greatergood.berkeley.edu/article/item/six_new_studies_that_can_help_you_rediscover_gratitude

https://research.com/education/scientific-benefits-of-gratitude

About the Author

Nathalie Herrey

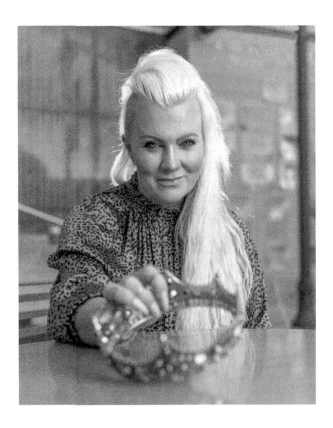

N athalie Herrey has had the opportunity to experience life in ways few can imagine - from excruciating hardship to finding joy! Today she lives her passion with a clear mission of helping others know that they can conquer anything life throws at them and claim their Crown. Life is meant to be lived with purpose, joy, and fulfillment.

With her degrees in Psychology and Leadership & Management, as well as decades as a corporate consultant, working with Tony Robbins,

Dean Graziosi, Jay Shetty, etc., along with her knowledge of social media, she has a passion for empowering men and women through servant leadership, providing them with tools and guidance to help them excel in their life and careers. Often using social media and personal/career branding, she helps them find and live their superpowers.

Her most outstanding achievement in life are her four children. She currently resides in Salt Lake City, UT, with her husband, four children, and three dogs. It is time to #StepIntoTheArena of your Life - it is time to #PickUpYourCrown 👑✨ https://www.nathalieherrey.com/

CHAPTER 9:
Beyond Flexibility:
The Unexpected Pathways of Self-Discovery

Yoga is more than just physical exercise; it's a powerful tool for self-discovery, personal growth, and inner peace. For the past seven years, I have been a petroleum engineer by day and a yoga teacher by night. Then, I pivoted from engineering to work for the university in corporate relations. Unfortunately, that did not work out, and I embraced and accepted the break from my career. It was tempting to prioritize binge-watching Netflix or having a pint of ice cream over taking care of myself because of life's daily pressures. So I embarked on a transformative 30-day yoga challenge to re-align and restore my energy. It opened my eyes to the endless possibilities within me, and I received more than I expected. I allowed myself to be vulnerable to all the emotions, and throughout the challenge, my heart opened to new possibilities for the next chapter of my journey. In this chapter, I want to inspire you by sharing the seven unexpected insights I discovered during this eye-opening experience.

Last March, I signed up for a 30-day limitless potential challenge. The rewards at first served as my motivation, and I was eager to experience the advantages of a regular yoga practice. Then, I set out to conquer the challenge and learn from various teachers. Finally, having never completed a yoga challenge, I was determined to make it happen this time.

And guess what? I succeeded! There were challenges in between throughout the practice, where I felt all the emotions I had set aside for quite some time. Who says it will be easy? And during practice, I permitted myself to let go — let go of the emotions, set free the expectations, and embrace all the feelings. Here are seven unexpected insights I gained during this transformative experience:

1. Gift of Presence - being in the moment. How often do we take a moment and be with our body or with people we love with full attention? Most of the time, we are all on our devices and do not pay attention. Throughout the challenge, I focused on being present and listening to my teacher's voice - my GPS throughout my practice. Being present helped me listen deeper to my body, leading to inward tuning.

2. Tuning into Yourself. Recognizing your body's unique needs is essential. Similar to being present, this is listening to what you need, what your body needs. Everyone's body is different, and listening to your body regardless of activity is essential. Know when to slow down, when to rest, and when to push your limits. For example, on the 7th day of yoga, I felt worn out and needed the rest, and instead of saying, "I am tired," I reviewed all the classes I'd taken. It was an AHA moment - most classes I took were power and needed a restore class. Because of slowing down and paying attention to my body, I knew what I needed - rest.

3. Move like no one is watching. Jump up, jump down, shake it up, sway your arms, swing your hips, and shake it out! It is your practice and no one else's. Although I am accustomed to structured yoga movements, I allowed myself to go with the flow and let go of my robotic moves. Through several days of practice doing this, I felt my energy shift. The energy shift occurred when I let go of what I thought I looked like to others. I owned up to what I needed - it is my practice.

4. Stillness. When was the last time you embraced silence or held a pose for more than one minute? Most of the time, we are so quick to move on to the next step or the next big thing in our lives that we miss out on the details of our journey. Instead, I learned to build up, add on, remove what was unnecessary, add back in, and see what works for me.

5. Breathe. Remember to breathe. Have you noticed that we sometimes hold our breath? It's common to hold our breath unconsciously, and proper breathing is essential in yoga, movement, and daily life. By focusing on our breath during each pose, we can experience a calming and soothing effect on our body and mind. Many yoga teachers, including me, emphasize the connection between breath and movement, encouraging practitioners to move mindfully and in sync with their breath. This practice helps us build a stronger sense of self-trust and harmony within ourselves.

6. Inner strength. Yoga is not only physical; it is mental. This aspect of yoga allowed me to slow down my thoughts and focus on the present moment, resulting in being mindful of my thoughts and feelings. With consistent practice and the combination of the first five things I learned, I gained more understanding of myself, emotional resilience, physical strength, and clarity of thought.

7. Change is constant. Everything around us changes every day. We change every day. My feelings today differ from how I feel tomorrow. We grow each day. Our movements, thoughts, and emotions are different, and it is okay.

The 30-day yoga challenge opened my eyes to the possibilities within myself. My experience with Kacie, one of my yoga teachers, allowed me to delve deeper into self-discovery. I realized how much my body needed this time to find myself again. I felt stuck in ways I did not imagine. I needed to listen to my body to find my way forward. Kacie helped me find the places where I was stuck. In her thought-provoking classes, her questions aligned with mine, pushing me to explore uncomfortable areas and decide whether to challenge myself physically or mentally. I needed it to regain my energy.

As a yoga teacher and a coach, I sometimes forget that I must replenish my cup to give more to my students. This challenge provided me with more than what I needed. I regained my physical strength and became mentally stronger, which allowed me to reconnect with myself. The unexpected insights were my guide to a transformative experience. This challenge is a testament to the incredible potential that lies within each of us. So, whether you're a seasoned yoga practitioner or a newbie, I encourage you to embrace the challenge, be present, and explore the depths of your being. Doing so will uncover an extraordinary world of self-awareness, acceptance, and inner strength that will profoundly impact your life. Remember, self-discovery is never-ending, and yoga offers a unique pathway to evolve and flourish continually. So embrace the practice and let the magic of yoga transform you on and off the mat.

About the Author

Regina Eco

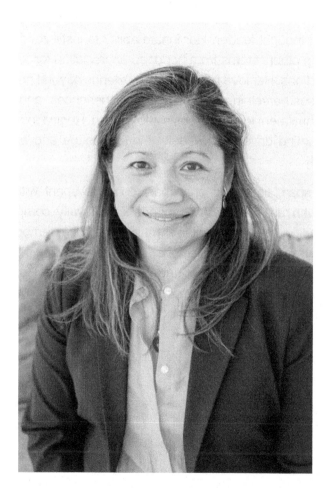

Regina Eco, a petroleum engineer with over 20 years of experience, has dedicated her career to energy, sustainability, continuous learning, and fostering strong relationships. As a strong believer in the power of connections, she consistently nurtures and values relationships in her personal and professional life.

Her professional accomplishments match her personal passions, which include being a lifelong athlete, yoga teacher, possibility coach, and travel enthusiast. Regina's devotion to mind-body balance has led her to teach yoga for eight years, enriching her life and sharing the benefits of mindfulness with others.

As a possibility coach, Regina empowers individuals to unlock their potential and overcome personal barriers, making her a sought-after mentor and thought leader. Her innate ability to instill confidence and motivation in others stems from her deep appreciation for relationships and connections. Her love for exploration extends beyond her career as she immerses herself in diverse cultures, experiences, and ideas that fuel her commitment to a more sustainable world. Regina's curiosity and love for learning drive her to seek new knowledge and experiences continuously.

In her spare time, she cherishes moments spent with her dog, Maverick, who reminds her of the importance of loyalty, companionship, and unconditional love. Regina's multifaceted life, embodying her professional achievements, personal interests, and dedication to the environment, inspires us all. Her unwavering commitment to a greener, more sustainable world demonstrates the power of passion, perseverance, and the value of building strong relationships.

https://www.radianceconsulting.co

https://www.linkedin.com/in/reginaeco

https://www.medium.com/@reginaeco

CHAPTER 10:
Touch is Essential for Growth, Healing from, and Preventing Generational and Physical Trauma

B oth our physical and emotional development and spiritual stability depend on safe and healthy human contact and connection. By nature, well-intended touch is essential; essential for well-being, growth, development, preventing faulty behaviors, and habitual survivalist mentalities. And not just a handshake or a hug once a year, but a habitual language embedded in our (at the very least) daily lives.

Being a licensed massage therapist specializing in professional and safe touch, it is heartbreaking to see how abusers warp touch and use it as a weapon to destroy the spirit and disrupt the trust and homeostasis of the body and mind. So much of individual and generational trauma's genesis derives from traumatic touch. When horrors like physical or sexual abuse take place (whether once or chronically), the epithelial cells spread the infectious lie to the victim's central nervous system that touch is abusive, harmful, unsafe, defiling, wicked, and, in a sense, murderous. Thus, the body becomes a grave with feelings of despair, shame, fury, hopelessness, and even dissociation that haunt like ghosts. Those ghosts cry out for various illnesses, disorders, and pathologies. When one's nature is distorted and severely abused, they develop aversions and, in a sense, allergies to what is naturally right and necessary for their own nature. And many, because of abuses and lack of consistent and loving touch, retreat and falsely protect with their possessed flight and fight tactics.

Furthermore, the body then remains in a constant state of fight or flight, torn between the earth and ground, the living (the present), and the dead (the past). A way to encourage healing from trauma and even prevent continuations of ancestral abuse even to preserve the wholesome nature of our future prosperity is touch: touch–human contact, skin-to-skin, hugs, and massage therapy. Touch is essential in healing and in preventing further tragedies in our everyday lives.

Infants without language have proved how our nervous systems and our livelihood's salvation depend on receiving continual loving and healthy touch. When we were infants, our cries to be held were the way to explain how vital physical touch was to our growth.

Furthermore, what ought to be taught differently is when we are not born with the aty/instinct to know how to self-soothe. Dr. Allan Schore is a leading expert in this psychological finding. The Right Orbital Frontal Cortex (ROFC) in the brain is where we regulate our limbic systems' survival reaction to stress, the area of our ability to calm down. During development in the womb and then through infancy, the infant learns how to self-soothe from their mother via their nervous system. The way to have direct access to the mother's nervous system is mainly lots of cuddles consumed with attentive and unconditional love.

If the infant's mother does not have a healthy nervous system, meaning she has anxiety or any other mental health issues, endured a lot of stress or mental illnesses during pregnancy and or postpartum, or is absent during their infancy, that child is predisposed to be incapable to self soothe and have healthy coping mechanisms. Though the child has never been punched or assaulted, that child will grow up living in a constant survival mode, fight, or flight mode, never relaxed or at ease, and in a continuous state of stress and physiological turmoil.

"Without having intensive, repeated, loving contact with the same one or two people, they simply can't make the proper connections."

The maternal nervous system imbalance would also imply that if the child is abused by the mother, the father, or any other person, the child's nervous system not only never learns how to self-soothe, but they are also designed and wired to self-protect and to separate from all they perceive as dangerous - touch. This is how parents, and soon-to-be parents, can be accountable now for breaking the generational abuses by prioritizing holding their children, no matter how old. We continue to rely on touch for our physical growth and emotional stability throughout our lives. Touch, the parental safe touch, is a necessary obligation to raise a stable generation.

So, what if you were not held and adored by your parents or even assaulted, and your nervous systems were corrupted by their or others' harmful manners? The way to help stop these fight or flight patterns and help restore rebalancing coping mechanisms is to interfere with the improper patterns with a healthy and safe touch from a grounded person with a healthy, calm nervous system. Though this is a parent's responsibility, this can come in the form of embrace from foster/adoptive parents, guardians, family members, and friends. Furthermore, such clients can also restore their nervous systems by receiving massage therapy.

The redemptive and curing benefits of massage therapy are irrefutable. The basic benefits of massage therapy include the prevention of diseases and injury, an increase in blood and lymphatic circulation, an increase in the exchange of nutrients, an increase in range of motion, a decrease in inflammation, and so many more redemptive properties. It is rarely discussed how massage therapy naturally increases levels of oxytocin, the hormone of bonding and connection, the same hormone that is naturally produced between mother and child after birth. Therefore, massage therapists provide a way for the client to learn how to trust through touch. This is where a professional relationship between the client and the massage therapist will build the support system needed for the client to break free from pasts that continue to torment the body and mind.

With clients that have carried physical trauma chronically, the more complex restorative properties of massage therapy show short-term benefits. Yet, some solutions and cures are long-term results of continual sessions along with psychotherapy. Massage therapy ignites the trigger points that activate the feelings entangled with them and commands them to speak, which may cause some triggering physical responses and overwhelming feelings of danger. This is where the massage therapist uses "resources" (the client's visualization of safe places or things that bring them peace and comfort) to prevent dissociating and firing up the nervous system with fear. Bringing breathwork into the touch therapy, calming and reprogramming the nervous system for peace by permitting safe and comforting touch to the body, massage therapy then brings the client present and interrupts the fight or flight tendencies.

This pattern, along with self-care routines and psychotherapy, will require time. But with commitment, trust, and hope for inner and somatic harmony, massage therapy can provide traumatized clients with a new hope for building upon safe and meaningful touch. Though massage is often pushed aside as merely a luxury, it is vital for mending the bonding and restoration process through safe and appropriate touch. The deficiency of wholesome interpersonal connection, communication, and touch is one we cannot afford to be deficient in. And it is a luxury that can be a remedy to traumatic experiences – showing the better and safer way of what should have been.

I have had many clients that have endured these kinds of sufferings, and most of the time, the physical and sexual trauma go hand in hand rather than apart. While some clients have been comfortable and even eager to receive the healing of touch, others are hesitant. It is essential that no matter what kind of trauma the client has endured, the client knows they are in a safe space, they have room to say no, and the healing process is not forced or rushed. With that given time, body tensions do melt into relaxation, emotional knots are washed away and calmed into peace, and fascia unwinds the muscles to receive proper circulation and strength. Massage permits clients to breathe easier, relearn proper postures, and, overall, their cells rewrite messages of empowerment through the gifts of massage therapy.

The body, mind, and spirit harmonies wither away with evil touch and the lack of righteous touch. Though traumatized bonding attachments encode falsehoods into our thoughts that we are better off without touch, it is irrevocably untrue. The human body, harmed or otherwise, aches for what our spirits long to feel, wholesome human contact. As we grow from childhood and even from conception, we embody core beliefs through our senses and what we perceive around us through our touch. If we are truly attended to and cared for by our parents and are fairly treated by those around us, we grow and succeed with our roots of healthy and tender touch. With the intentions of compassion, kindness, relief, support, soothing, and peace (all being pure and safe), you can heal one's misdirected aversions with touch. Touch melts—touch releases. Touch purifies. Touch heals. To feel is to heal; we replace our body's cells that have been tainted by the fingerprints of the wicked with nourished cells that have received cuddles and hugs and are filled with affection and, additionally, by regularly receiving supportive massage therapy.

About the Author

Sariah Boyer

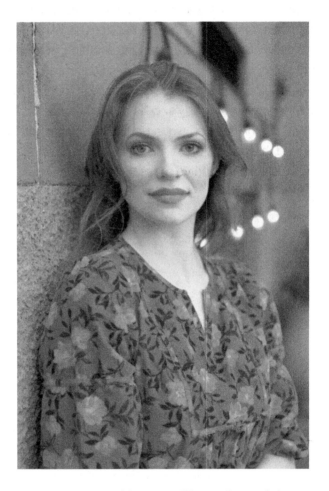

S ariah Boyer is a Licensed Massage Therapist and the owner of Mother and Mine Massage in Draper, Utah. Sariah witnesses the healing power of touch and massage therapy regarding healing from traumatic events. She went into massage therapy school four days after her high school graduation and has been a massage therapist since 2019. She has seen many clients that have/continue to suffer from their past traumatic experiences mentally and physically. Her purpose and designs with her business are to help build up a part of "the village" for mothers. She helps mothers and children create healing bonds, heal women and mothers and transform from their trauma through all intended safe, comforting, supportive, healthy, and kind touch – massage therapy. She is pursuing her Infant Massage Certification and her Trauma Touch Certification to help establish those purposes.

Sariah is a wife to Jonathan, another Licensed Massage Therapist, and a mother to her sweet and free-spirited daughter, Sally.

You can find more about her and Mother and Mine Massage at motherandminemassage.com

@motherandminemassage Instagram and Facebook

CHAPTER 11:
Human Design: The Story of You

In oneself lies the whole world, and if you know how to look and learn, the door is there, and the key is in your hand. Nobody on earth can give you either the key or the door to open, except yourself." —Jidda Krishnamurti.

I can't remember how Human Design fell into my lap, but I remember the first time I read my chart, which is generated using your birth date, birth time, and birthplace. Back then, I didn't know what I was looking at as a whole. I simply looked up one thing at a time.

With each bit of information, my shoulders dropped as I discovered more about myself. I sighed in relief, and at some point, I started crying. I remember thinking, "I'm not broken. There's nothing wrong with me. I'm just me."

It was validating. It was my permission slip to embrace who I am at the core fully. To follow my inner knowing and to step into my truth.

Not that I needed permission, none of us do, but I had been living my life in an internal struggle between *what I felt was true for me* and the story I was living in *who I thought I needed to be.*

That story was created through conditioning.

Conditioning is learned behavior patterns created around the meanings we've given to and in response to thoughts, beliefs, trauma, memories, life experiences, genetic conditioning, ancestral lineage, and emotional artifacts of everything that's ever happened to you.

Our perception of the world and the meanings we hold influence what we create in life.

For example, as a child, your mother constantly criticized you (thinking she was building character), which led to creating protective behaviors, such as agreeing with her instead of speaking your mind, working yourself to the bone to get a 5.0 GPA, or going to college for accounting rather than art.

These seemingly harmless childhood protective behaviors create your narrative as a people pleaser. People pleasing can negatively affect every area of your life as an adult leading to a marriage that isn't profoundly fulfilling, a soul-sucking career path, living out patterns that keep you from believing you can have what you really want in life, allowing everyone around you to walk all over you, and living in pure exhaustion.

The story you've been trying to keep up with your whole life may not really be YOUR story. Human Design allows you to see where you're creating a reality that isn't right for you.

It shows you your potential in its highest and lowest form. Using the example above, Human Design shines Light on people-pleasing behavioral patterning (lowest form), and it shows you that there's another option for you to be a sovereign human being who takes control of her destiny (highest form) and what that looks like.

You are the happiest and most abundant when you're creating in alignment with the highest expression of you and your unique energy blueprint. Human Design opens your eyes to the full potential of who you can be and gives you new language to change your narrative.

The Human Design system synthesizes spirituality and ancient and modern sciences—astrology, I Ching, Kabbalah, biochemistry, genetics, the chakra system, Vedic Philosophy, and quantum physics.

It uses two astrological metrics; the Human Design chart shows planetary alignment at your birth time (conscious/Personality) and planetary position at 88 degrees, or three months, before birth (unconscious/Design).

Human Design has five Types: Manifestor, Generator, Projector, Reflector, and Manifesting Generator. Each of these Types tells you who you are, what you're here to do, and how you will do it. Manifestors make up roughly 9% of the world's population and are here to get the ball rolling. They're the initiators and inventors and operate through deep bursts of creative energy and rest cycles. Generators are the world's workhorses and makeup roughly 30% of the entire population. Projectors make up approximately 20% of the world's population. These are the Seers, and they offer wisdom and guidance to the rest of the world. Reflectors make up roughly 1% of the world's population. They can make great leaders. They have no consistent energy of their own—they reflect the energy of their environment. Manifesting Generators make up roughly 40% of the world's population and are a hybrid between Manifestors and Generators.

Your Strategy is the unique way you make decisions, interact with others, and take action in the world.

Your Profile, derived from the I-Ching hexagram line expressions in your Sun and Earth placements, from both sides of the chart—Design/unconscious and Personality/conscious—and gives you insight into the character you play in the story and describes your characteristics, social, investigative, experimental, hermit, projective, or a role model.

Your Incarnation Cross is made up of the Sun and Earth I Ching hexagrams, or Gates, from both sides of the chart—Design/unconscious and Personality/conscious—and is the plot outline of your story. It's the cornerstone of your life purpose.

Human Design is a roadmap, a guide, and a tool for human understanding. It reflects who you are as a unique, one-of-a-kind powerful human being.

It tells you how you experience the world, how you process information, how you best make decisions, how to navigate relationships, how to live out your purpose, and how to live in harmony with your authentic Self. It's a tool for rewriting the story of you.

Your Human Design chart is the code of your life story, who you truly came here to be, and your soul curriculum. The more true to your Design you live, the more you can be in the full expression of the Light that is YOU, the real you. The road to living your happiest, most fulfilled Self is not a one-size-fits-all template. It's unique to only YOU. Human Design helps you recognize your innate gifts to be who you truly came here to be, which is the simplest way to live your dream life.

About the Author

Tina LeAnn

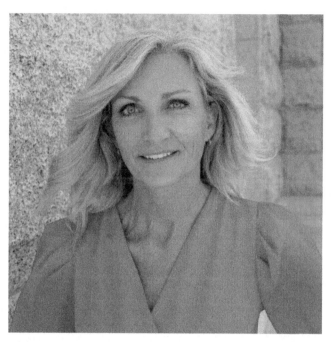

Tina LeAnn is a 3/5 Emotional Manifestor who intuitively lives her Design through experimenting with life and sharing her findings in service of humanity. She's traveled the world, trekked to Mount Everest Basecamp, summited Mt. Kilimanjaro, and most recently spent a year living as a nomad while driving a 1971 Plymouth Cuda.

It was in that literal and metaphorical vehicle of transformation where she found true joy, regained her life force energy, and came home to herself. Upon reflection, she discovered focused codes within the Human Design Chart that, when unraveled, inadvertently loosen the grip on many other energetic knots.

Tina wholeheartedly believes that the human body is the key to the Kingdom. It is through human technology, heart coherence, and love of Self where we find a deep connection to a Divine Source.

https://www.tinaleann.co/

https://www.facebook.com/webdesignbadassery

CHAPTER 12:
Unlock The Power of Your Authenticity

"What you think, you become." – Siddhartha Gautama Buddha.

Your thoughts drive your emotions. When you change your thoughts, you change your emotions. But what about the times you react intensely, without even thinking? In those situations, it feels like your brain is shutting down and you're being "triggered". These intense emotional reactions can be the result of a past traumatic experience that needs healing. I refer to these as "feeling memories."

We first experience everything in the world with our five senses – our sight, hearing, taste, smell, and touch. Our sensory experiences are stored in the limbic system of the brain, specifically the Hippocampus. The limbic system is considered our survival brain, the seat of our emotions and motivation, and is involved in the processing of memories. (3) Memories and experiences are cataloged by the Hippocampus and distributed to other areas of the brain that use language for easier retrieval later.

Not all memories are stored the same. Traumatic memories – events that evoke intense emotions – are sent to the amygdala,(2) your protector brain, and are not cataloged by the Hippocampus or distributed. Trauma is not the event itself but our body's response to a set of circumstances. Your protector brain does not use language and doesn't tell time. (1) It can't tell the difference between you being five years old and thirty-five. When activated, your protector brain has four ways of protecting you – run, fight, play dead, or people please. As odd as it may seem, excessive people-pleasing is actually considered a trauma response.

We all want to have the approval and acceptance of others. However, people pleasers go to the extreme of prioritizing others' needs and wants to the point of exhaustion, completely losing their own identity. They become trapped in a cycle of self-devaluation and struggle to notice their personal strengths.

How do you clear these "feeling memories" from your body?

You heal them through your body. Through your senses. What is your body trying to tell you?

You are not broken. It's not all in your head. It's in your body.

We remember past intensely emotional experiences with body sensations and feelings before language. What are your body's "feeling memories"?

When these "feeling memories" are not released, your body becomes trained to live in a state of alert for long periods. You can feel anxious, sad, confused, unable to relax or sleep, and exhausted. You might experience feeling like you are in a fog, have an overall sense of numbness, and feel disconnected from the world.

Your body is your oldest, wisest friend who has wonderful wisdom to share with you when you learn how to listen. Somatic body processing or "body mindfulness" is the fastest way to process emotions, thoughts, or physical sensations. Little or no language is needed. "Body mindfulness" eliminates the need to tell the story about the intensely emotional past experience.

Learn to harness your true potential and unlock the power of your authenticity.

Prioritizing authenticity and embracing your true self is crucial for personal growth and fulfillment. Living a life that aligns with your values and beliefs allows you to experience a sense of genuine happiness and fulfillment.

However, freeing your authenticity can be challenging and scary. It often requires breaking away from societal expectations and overcoming social conditioning.

Remember, embracing your authenticity is an ongoing process. It requires continuous self-reflection, self-acceptance, and the willingness to live authentically, even in the face of challenges. By prioritizing your authentic self, you can lead a more fulfilling and rewarding life that is true to who you are.

A woman, let's call her Melody, reached out to me for help resolving a conflict she was having with her son and daughter-in-law. Melody was heartbroken because she was not able to have a relationship with her grandchildren and wanted a more fulfilling connection with her son.

Melody felt like a failure, had a habit of apologizing often, was overly involved in the feelings of others, wondered if she was just being "overly sensitive", and would do almost anything to avoid confrontation. She held back her authentic self from her son and others out of fear of rejection or losing the relationship completely.

First, I helped Melody step out of her story about the situation and get clear on what she was feeling. Then, we were able to craft how to express to her son what she needed in a way that he could truly understand. Next, I showed her how to stop putting herself last and move past the guilty feelings that surfaced when she tried taking care of herself. She began to experience more joy and happiness in her life. By unlocking the power of her authenticity, Melody was able to know her worthiness, express how she felt clearly to others, ask for what she needed, and confidently decide when something was a yes or a no for her. The relationship with her son improved, all because she worked on herself and healed her "feeling memories".

If, like Melody, you struggle with losing yourself in relationships, have no idea who you are, or are second-guessing yourself, please know you're not alone. There is support for you.

I can help you show up and speak up unapologetically in all areas of your life.

By showing you how to access your inner strengths and cultivate healthy love for yourself, I will teach you to unlock the power of your authenticity and shift you from stuck to fulfilled.

If you're tired of putting everyone else's needs before your own, it's time to take action. Learn to harness your true potential and unlock the power of living your most authentic, inspired life. Don't wait any longer to start living the life you deserve! May you find peace, love, and happiness as you find your way back to you.

About the Author

Tina Jones

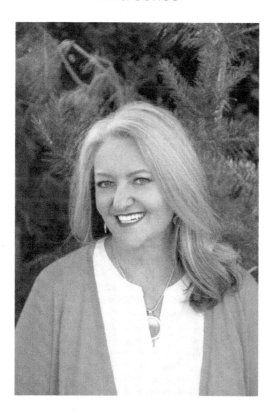

Tina Jones is passionate about facilitating breakthroughs in others' lives. She moves her clients out of stress, anxiety, or mood swings into confidence, courage, and emotional balance. She can quickly diffuse conflict situations and will show you how to stand in your personal power even in the face of difficult people or situations.

She walks her talk and shares real-life experiences as she teaches. Clients call Tina relatable, entertaining, and engaging. Her style of facilitation makes her "hands-on" workshops worth every penny. During her 25 years as an entrepreneur, she has built multiple businesses, from idea to execution to sale.

When not transforming lives, Tina can be found dancing in the kitchen to her favorite tunes, hiking a river trail, or experimenting with new abstract art techniques.

Facebook: https://www.facebook.com/tinajones.net/

Instagram: https://www.instagram.com/tinajones_empoweryou/

Website: https://www.tinajones.net/

About the Author

Susana Perez

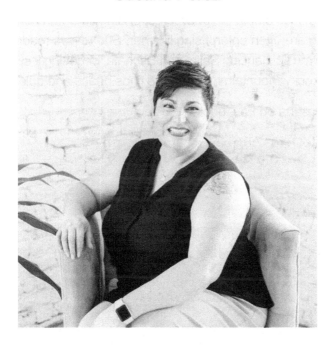

Susana Perez is a #1 International Bestselling Author and the founder of Creativo Publishing, LLC, a boutique full-service firm that specializes in premium author services specifically designed for busy professionals. Our end-to-end services include writer coaching, ghostwriting, editing, proofing, cover design, book layout, eBook production, Audiobook production, marketing, and Bestseller strategy.

Susana Pérez is an Author, Publisher, Mentor, and Coach. She emigrated to the US in 2001, speaking little English. She started her first company in 1998, a printing service serving small and medium-sized companies in Montevideo, Uruguay. Susana is a dynamic and enthusiastic entrepreneur who has worked in the areas of advertising, customer service, sales, graphic design, cleaning, and food industries.

She connects with her audience through her unique approach to business and life, her sense of humor, her business skills, and her sincere interest in her client's success. She inspires her clients to maximize their influence, achieve their goals, and ultimately, impact everyone they encounter.

Susana finds a balance between spending time with her family and friends who are often enterprising like her. She enjoys reading, writing, listening to music, dancing Salsa and Bachata, or getting lost in the trails of Utah's Rocky Mountains, where she finds peace and quiet.

Find Susana on Facebook: www.facebook.com/susana.perez.us

Website: https://thebestsellermaker.com/

Made in the USA
Middletown, DE
19 August 2023